PRETTY
AS A
PEACH

First published in Great Britain, Australia and New Zealand in 2018
by Modern Books

An imprint of Elwin Street Productions Limited
14 Clerkenwell Green
London EC1R 0DP
www.modern-books.com

ISBN 978-1-911130-78-9

10 9 8 7 6 5 4 3 2 1

Printed in China

PRETTY
AS A
PEACH

*Janet Hayward and
Susie Prichard-Casey*

Illustrations by
Arielle Gamble

(m)

JANET HAYWARD has over 15 years' experience in the beauty and cosmetics industry and is the co-founder of the beauty and health website, beautydirectory.com.au, which is followed by beauty experts worldwide. She is the author of *Lemons Are a Girl's Best Friend*. Originally from the United Kingdom Janet now lives in Sydney, Australia with her family.

SUSIE PRICHARD-CASEY is a natural beauty and body guru who holds advanced diplomas in Remedial Massage, Reflexology and LaStone Therapy. Susie has worked for Neal's Yard amongst other top UK spas. Susie lives in Berkshire, England where she keeps bees and is developing her own honey and organic product range.

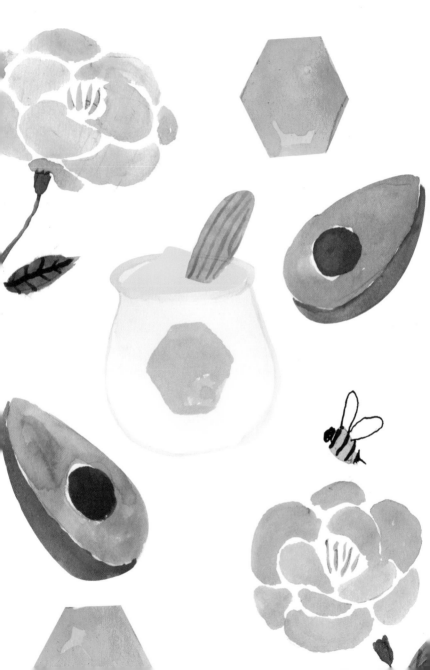

CONTENTS

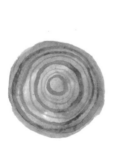
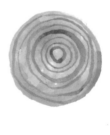

HOW TO GET YOUR GLOW

Beauty is enjoying an artisanal revival with many beauty lovers turning to traditional and natural ingredients to indulge in personalized hair treatments, body creams and bespoke facial products. Unlike mass-produced versions, these pamper products and treatments can be customized to work wonders on the body, mind and soul.

For best results with these treatment recipes, wherever possible always choose organically-grown options for raw ingredients to ensure integrity and efficacy. Organic ingredients have been nurtured without the addition of chemical fertilisers or other growth-promoters and have also been processed without the addition of chemicals, in order to retain the essence of the ingredient as nature intended.

Preparation is key to ensure the best results, so before you embark on the creation of your own beauty products, it's a good idea to gather together the recipe ingredients and specified utensils and vessels ready on the kitchen bench. Whether you are making a face mask, moisturizer or a bath soak, ensure you have pre-sterilized the jars or bottles so they are waiting ready to pour or spoon in your freshly made beauty preparations.

GENERAL PREPARATION EQUIPMENT

Most of the equipment you need to make the beauty products in this book are regular kitchen utensils and vessels. There is no need to buy special equipment although you may need to stock up on a selection of wooden spoons and spatulas as these can absorb the scents of some of the preparations. The following list is a general guide to what you might need to make any of the products:

- Glass bowls (large and small) for mixing
- Measuring jug
- Measuring spoons
- Weighing scales
- Saucepans (different sizes)
- Wooden spoons
- Soft spatula
- Glass droppers (pipettes)
- Blender/Food Processor
- Whisk
- Funnel

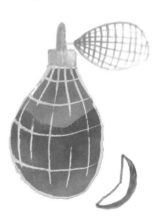

BUYING INGREDIENTS

Many of the base ingredients used in these recipes can be found in a kitchen store cupboard – for example, bicarbonate of soda, olive oil, sea salt, etc. As with cooking, best results come from the best ingredients and always weigh or measure according to the suggested method. Wherever possible use organically sourced ingredients to limit the presence of unwanted chemicals.

Health food stores and good supermarkets are the best sources of organic base ingredients such as coconut oil, olive oil, sea salt, oats, honey, etc. Local farmers' markets and garden centres are great suppliers of organically-grown fruits and vegetables plus fresh herbs and flowers that feature in some of the recipes.

Essential oils and tinctures are best sourced from health food stores, some pharmacies or specialist suppliers that can confirm the provenance and are more readily able to guarantee organic authenticity and quality. Many of these suppliers can be found online with good testimonials.

TECHNIQUE HACKS

The beauty recipes in the book have easy-to-follow methods for preparation; however, it's always handy to have a short-cut tip! In cold weather, coconut oil is solid and harder to use in some recipes. To transform it to liquid form, simply scoop the required amount of coconut oil into a glass bowl and stand over hot water. This removes the possibility of overheating or burning the oil.

If a recipe requires a small quantity of an essential oil, practice using a dropper with water into a spare bowl before adding the essential oil to a recipe. There is an art to getting the pressure correct to ensure only a single drop falls into the preparation. When adding honey to a recipe, always warm the spoon under the hot tap first to ensure the honey runs freely from the spoon and into your beauty preparation.

Patch test

As with all personal care and beauty products, it is always best to patch test a small amount of the product on the underside of your arm for an allergic reaction before using a large quantity of the product on your skin.

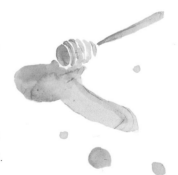

STORING YOUR BEAUTY PRODUCTS

Choosing different jars and bottles for your beauty products takes product personalization to the next level, especially if you are making the products for gifts. Glass is always the best option for storage – it is easy to clean and also recyclable. If your recipe is high in essential oils, the quality of the finished product will be retained for longer by storing it in coloured glass to protect it from sunlight.

You can re-use empty jars and pots that once held your favourite lotions and potions but do take care to wash them thoroughly to remove any leftover product and aromas.

To get started it's a good idea to have a small stock of the following:

You will need:

glass jars with screw top lids, small and large •
glass bottles with screw top lids • glass spray bottles •
sticky label and a pen

To prepare:

Notes are included with each recipe to advise shelf life and special storage tips but all freshly made beauty products are best kept out of direct sunlight and preferably in the fridge.

SAFETY NOTES AND PRECAUTIONS

Before handling any ingredients, be sure to wash your hands thoroughly and sterilize tools with boiling water to eliminate bacteria that could contaminate your products.

To sterilize the jars, bottles, pots and sprays, place them in the dishwasher – lids off and on a separate shelf – and run through the hottest wash. Allow them to air-dry, using a paper towel to mop up any excess water to reduce the risk of contamination, then replace the lids.

Always test the product on a small area of skin first and take care when applying any treatment to the sensitive eye area. If you experience any itching or redness, rinse the affected area with clean water immediately.

The recipes do not contain the chemical preservatives that are found in store-bought items therefore not all products will keep well for a period of time. Do take care to stick to the quantity and storage advice given for each recipe.

It is best to store products that will keep in the fridge, as indicated with the recipe. Always use a spatula or a spoon to transfer your products to sterilized containers.

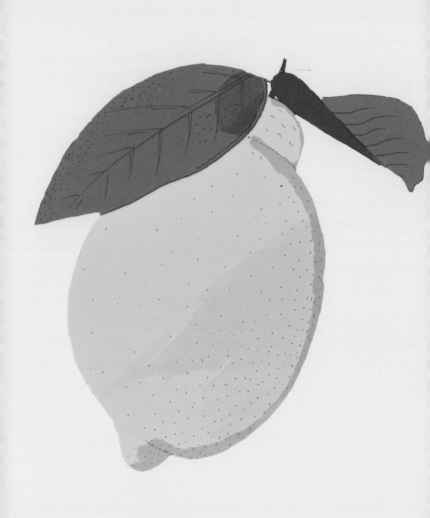

FRUIT

With ingredients including cleansing apple, brightening strawberries, nourishing banana and vitamin-packed peach, these recipes contain delicious nutrients for soft skin, fabulous hair and happy hands and nails.

STRAWBERRY BRIGHTEN UP

This face mask will help restore tone and vitality to your skin. Strawberries add colour to your skin, as their antioxidants help to fight free radicals, which may rob the skin of its luster. Cucumber is also extremely cooling. This mask is ideal for all skin types. You can apply honey directly to spots or scars to help speed up the healing process.

You will need:

1 tablespoon ground almonds • 3 strawberries • ½ cucumber • 1 teaspoon honey • 1 tablespoon yoghurt

To prepare:

Blend the ingredients together until smooth.

To use:

Apply the mixture to cleansed, damp skin. Leave for 15 minutes or until dry. Gently wipe off with a damp wash cloth.

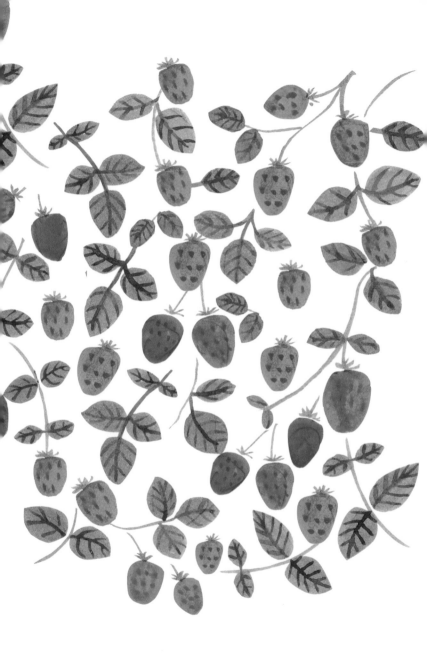

TOMATO AND MILK JUICE CLEANSER

The high acid content in the recipe – lactic acid in the milk and fruit acid in the tomato – gives this lotion a gentle peeling action. Test on the inside arm or wrist for any possible allergic reactions before using on the face. Recommended for both normal and oily skin types.

You will need:

1 medium very ripe tomato • 150 ml fresh whole milk • filtered water

To prepare:

Juice or blend the tomato. Strain through a piece of muslin or tea towel, and discard the pulp. Add the tomato juice to an equal amount of fresh milk.

To use:

Apply to the face and neck, using cotton pads, once or twice a day. Leave on for 10 minutes and rinse with filtered water and pat dry. Store in a covered container or bottle in the fridge. Keep for no longer than five days.

BRIGHTENING FRUIT FACIAL

Perfect for all skin types, this facial can be tailored for the best results by selecting an astringent fruit for use with oily skin or a soothing one for dry to sensitive skin. Make fresh each time.

You will need:

6 tablespoons milk powder • 1 tablespoon honey • for your preferred fruit choose from; 1 medium-sized banana for dry to sensitive skin; 6 strawberries for oily skin

To prepare:

Mash the banana or the strawberries in a small bowl and then add the milk powder and honey. Mix together until all the ingredients are thoroughly combined.

To use:

Smooth all over your face and neck using fingertips and leave for at least 10 minutes for the best results. Remove the mask with tissues before rinsing your face with warm water.

STRAWBERRY FACIAL STEAMER

A fragrant facial steamer to refresh your pores and perfectly prep your skin for your favourite facial oil or moisturizer.

You will need:
4 strawberries • 2 camomile teabags

To prepare:
Make two cups of camomile tea and leave to infuse for 5 minutes. Mash the strawberries in a mixing bowl, then pour in the tea. Pour boiling water over the mixture to the half-full level of the bowl. Leave to stand for 3 minutes.

To use:
Lean over the bowl, with your face at least 20 cm away from the water level, and cover your head with a towel. Keep your eyes and mouth closed and breathe in the fragrance. After 5 minutes, remove the towel and splash your face with cool water to close the pores.

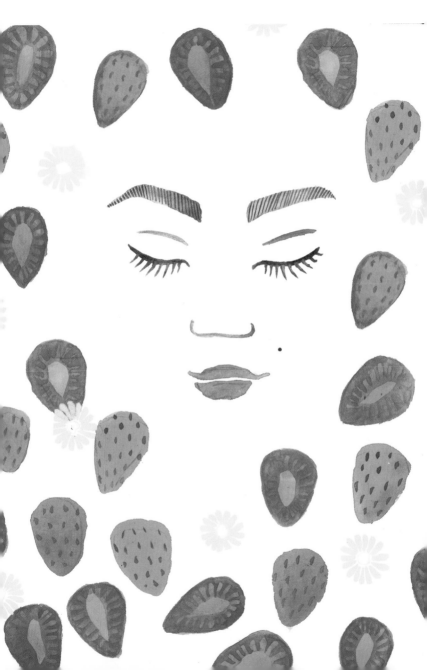

FRESH WATERMELON MASK

Watermelon is extremely refreshing and very hydrating for the skin. This recipe is excellent for oily skin. If you have dry skin, add a banana instead of yoghurt.

You will need:

100 g watermelon, chopped • 3 tablespoons yoghurt

To prepare:

Mash the watermelon in a small bowl until smooth. Add the yoghurt and blend.

To use:

Apply to the face and neck, and cover your face with a moist cloth. Leave for 10 minutes and rinse with lukewarm water. Rinse dry.

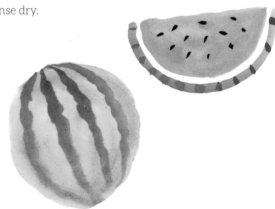

ANTI-AGEING BANANA MASK

Bananas contain large quantities of magnesium, potassium, iron, zinc, iodine and vitamins A, B, E and F. This mask is an ideal anti-ageing treatment for skin of all ages.

You will need:

1 small banana • 2 tablespoons fresh heavy cream • 1 tablespoon honey • 1 tablespoon oat flour • bottled or spring water

To prepare:

Mash the banana, then add cream, honey and flour. Mix well. You may need to add more cream or flour to obtain the right consistency.

To use:

Apply mask to a clean face, making sure you include the area around the eyes and the neck, and leave on for 30 minutes. Rinse off with water and pat dry.

CITRUS BODY WASH

This zesty lemon body wash is a great way to wake up the senses during a morning shower.

You will need:

4 tablespoons liquid Castile soap • glass jar with lid • 1 tablespoon honey • 1 tablespoon jojoba oil • 20 drops of lemon essential oil • 5 drops of spearmint essential oil • 4 vitamin E capsules

To prepare:

Pour the liquid Castile soap into the glass jar and add the honey, jojoba oil, lemon essential oil and spearmint essential oil. Swirl to mix, then break open and add the vitamin E capsules.

To use:

Screw on the lid and shake well to combine the ingredients. Pour a little body wash onto a loofah and enjoy the lather's cleansing, moisturising properties.

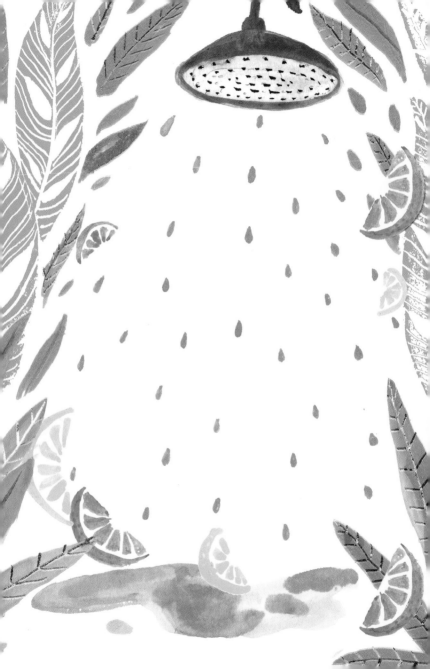

RED-BERRY POWDER BLUSH

This natural blush offers buildable colour, so you can choose a light blush or apply more for a stronger evening look.

You will need:

2 tablespoons arrowroot flour • 1 teaspoon red-berry powder • raw cacao powder (optional) • small pot with a lid

To prepare:

Sieve the arrowroot flour into a small glass bowl and then slowly add the red-berry powder and mix. Test the colour with a tiny pinch of the powder mix on the back of the hand until the desired shade is achieved. If the colour becomes too pink, add a little of the cacao powder to deepen the final shade. Once mixed, spoon into a small pot and it's ready.

To use:

Swirl a little of the powder on the apples of your cheeks with a blusher brush and slowly add more to build your perfect, healthy glow.

PEACH, ROSE WATER AND LEMON FACE MASK FOR OILY, BLEMISHED SKIN

Rich in folates, peaches replenish and boost cellular renewal, as their natural vitamin E content helps restore skin and can assist in reducing blemishes, such as acne scarring.

You will need:

½ ripe peach • ½ lemon • 1 teaspoon rose water

To prepare:

Purée the peach in a food processor to a fine paste. Place in a glass bowl and add the lemon juice and rose water. Mix well.

To use:

Apply with fingertips to the face and neck, avoiding the eye area and leave for 20 minutes. Rinse gently in warm water and pat dry. Skin will feel fresh and thoroughly clean.

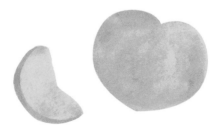

LEMON NAIL WHITENER

Regular nail polish wearers will understand the issue of yellowing nails. Restore a fresh, clean look with this whitening treatment that can be used weekly. Make fresh each time.

You will need:

juice of ½ lemon • 2 teaspoons bicarbonate soda

To prepare:

Mix the lemon juice with the bicarbonate soda in a small bowl. Apply this paste to each fingernail and massage gently to remove stains.

To use:

Rinse with warm water, gently pat dry, then treat nails to a massage with Shea Nut Butter Cuticle Cream (page 125).

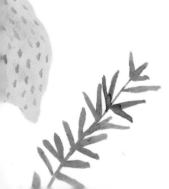

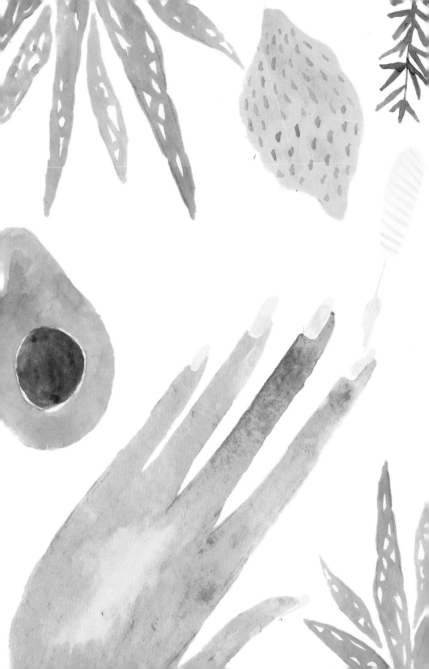

SKIN TIGHTENING PEACH AND EGG WHITE FACE MASK

Egg white nourishes and helps to both tighten and firm skin as well as pores, smoothing fine lines and wrinkles for a fresh, youthful complexion. A quick and easy recipe that gives glowing results.

You will need:

½ ripe peach • 1 egg white

To prepare:

Place the peach and egg white into a food processor and blend to a fine paste.

To use:

Cleanse skin then apply to the face and neck with the fingertips, excluding the sensitive eye and under-eye areas. Leave for 20-30 minutes then rinse with warm water and pat dry.

DETOXIFYING GREEN CLAY AND PEACH FACE MASK

Great for all skin types, green clay is high in minerals and is a powerful detoxifier. The avocado and peaches act to soften and moisturize, boosting cell regeneration and promoting skin elasticity. Excellent for acne scars, breakouts and patchy skin.

You will need:

2 tablespoons French green clay powder • 2 tablespoons avocado • 2 tablespoons peach

To prepare:

Mash the avocado and peach together in a glass bowl before adding the clay powder. Stir well to form a fine paste.

To use:

Cleanse skin and then, using fingertips, apply the paste to the face and neck, avoiding the eye area. Leave for 20 minutes then tissue off residue and rinse gently with warm water and pat dry.

ENERGIZING FACE PACK

For optimal effect, try using a gentle facial scrub before applying the face pack and finish with a nourishing facial treatment oil.

You will need:

25 g green clay powder • 1 teaspoon cornflour • 1 egg yolk • 1 teaspoon brewer's yeast • 1 teaspoon jojoba oil • 1 drop of geranium essential oil

To prepare:

Combine the green clay and cornflour, and mix well. Add the egg yolk, brewer's yeast and jojoba oil, and add to the powder to form a smooth paste. Add the geranium oil and re-mix.

To use:

Apply the mixture to the face and leave for 15 minutes. Remove with warm water and gently pat dry. Make fresh each time and use once a week for best results.

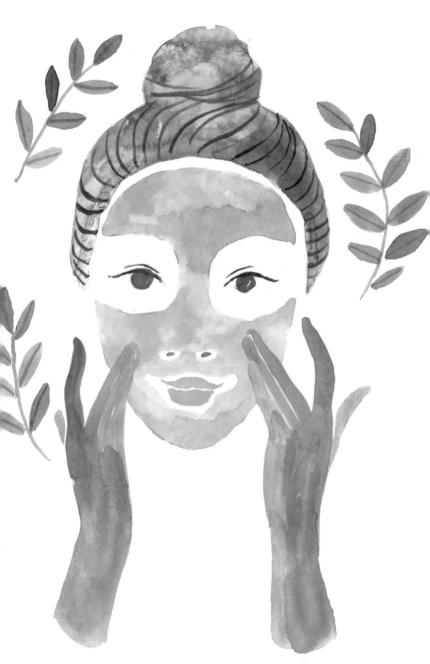

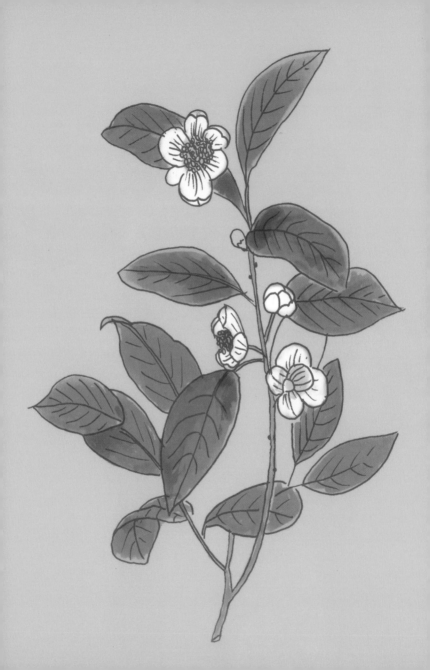

FLOWERS & HERBS

Gentle rose, purifying parsley, soothing lavender and brightening camomile all make flowers and herbs the perfect choice for anyone wanting to pamper skin, body and hair whilst invigorating the senses with these intoxicating scents.

CAMOMILE HAIR RINSE

The effects of this quick and easy hair rinse are cumulative, so be sure to use this regularly for a gradual lightening effect.

You will need:

6–8 camomile teabags • freshly boiled water

To prepare:

Steep the teabags in 1 litre of boiling water for 30 minutes to make a good, strong brew. Transfer the tea into a jug and add about 1 litre of cool water to make a diluted solution.

To use:

With your head over a large bowl in a basin or sink, slowly pour the diluted brew through the hair. For short hair, the solution can be spritzed into the hair with a dispenser bottle for ease. Comb through to the ends, then pour the liquid back into the jug and repeat the rinsing and combing process three times. Allow the hair to absorb the final camomile rinse by wrapping a towel around the head for 30 minutes before rinsing with warm water.

GRAPESEED AND BORAGE OIL CLEANSER

Borage oil is rich in skin-loving gamma-linoleic acids that help soothe sensitive, inflamed or reactive skin and leaves skin feeling clean and smooth.

You will need:

30 ml glass dropper bottle • grapeseed oil • borage oil • 10 drops of essential oil, choose from: camomile, to calm sensitive skin; lavender, to heal skin, especially acne scars; rose, to improve texture and tone • clean cotton face cloth

To prepare:

Fill the glass bottle two-thirds full with grapeseed oil. Add enough borage oil to fill the bottle and then add your chosen essential oil. Screw the top on the bottle and shake to blend.

To use:

To thoroughly clean your face and neck, use your fingers to massage in 3 drops of the cleanser, then use a damp cotton face cloth to gently wipe away the dust and grime of the day. Use morning and night.

ROSE BATH MILK

This rose bath milk will leave your skin feeling soft and moisturized, and your mind relaxed, thanks to the Epsom salts and oils.

You will need:

30 ml glass dropper bottle • grapeseed oil • borage oil • 10 drops of essential oil, choose from: camomile, to calm sensitive skin; lavender, to heal skin, especially acne scars; rose, to improve texture and tone • clean cotton face cloth

To prepare:

Combine the milk powder with the Epsom salts in a glass bowl, then add the rose essential oil and dried rose petals. Mix together thoroughly, then seal in an airtight container.

To use:

Run a warm bath and drop in a handful of the bath mixture. Step into the luxurious, silky bath for the ultimate in relaxation.

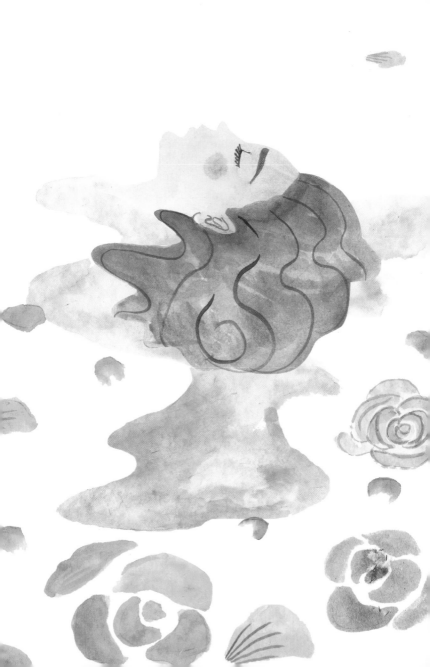

HOT CLOTH COCONUT AND ROSE WATER CLEANSING BALM

The perfect, beautifully scented cleansing balm with rose
water to sweep away everyday grime and soothe irritation.
Antimicrobial coconut oil helps melt away make-up, adding
antioxidant nourishment to leave skin hydrated and soft.

You will need:

10 ml rose water • 3 tablespoons coconut oil • muslin
face cloth

To prepare:

Mix the coconut oil with the rose water in a glass bowl, then
transfer to a small glass jar with a lid. Place in the fridge.

To use:

Scoop a generous amount of the cleansing balm into the
hand and warm between the fingers. Massage gently all
over the face, including the eye area, to loosen impurities
and dissolve make-up. Rinse the muslin cloth in hot water.
Squeeze out the water and use the hot, damp cloth to gently
sweep away the balm. Take care not to burn your skin!

CORIANDER COMPLEXION TREAT

A night-time, detoxifying and exfoliating treatment that offers an antioxidant boost. Coriander is a powerhouse herb that is full of minerals and vitamin C.

You will need:

½ bunch of coriander • 2 teaspoons of natural yoghurt • 1 teaspoon lemon juice • 1 tablespoon honey

To prepare:

Grind the coriander with a pestle and mortar to retain the juice and the pulp, then transfer to a glass bowl. Add the yoghurt, lemon juice and honey and stir until thoroughly mixed.

To use:

Apply to the face, avoiding the eye area, then relax and leave for 15 minutes. Rinse away in cool water and skin will look clear, revitalized and will feel beautifully smooth.

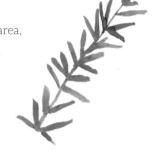

COCONUT AND LAVENDER BODY CREAM

Nourish all skin, even sensitive types, with this super-hydrating ointment. Lavender oil revitalizes the skin and its antiseptic properties help to clear up acne and other blemishes.

You will need:
250 ml coconut oil • 4 drops of lavender oil • glass jar with lid

To prepare:
Melt the coconut oil in a glass bowl over a saucepan of boiling water. Add the lavender oil and combine thoroughly, then remove from the heat.

Allow to cool and firm up, until almost solid. Then, using a hand blender or manual whisk, beat the mixture until it becomes light and creamy. Spoon into the jar and seal, ready to use.

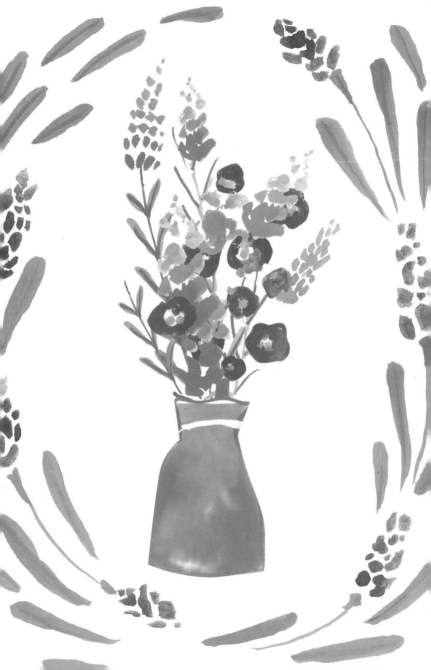

GREEN TEA CLEANSER

Rich in polyphenols, a powerful antioxidant, green tea helps to reduce the free radicals that can cause premature ageing.

You will need:

2 teaspoons green tea leaves • spring water, freshly boiled • 5 drops of jojoba oil • cotton wool pads

To prepare:

Place the green tea leaves in a small, clean cup and pour in 5 tablespoons of spring water. Leave to steep for 5 minutes. Strain the tea into a small bowl and stir in the jojoba oil.

To use:

Dip a cotton wool pad into the cleanser and sweep over your face, repeating with a clean cotton wool pad until the cleanser is used up. Use morning and night. Prepare fresh each time.

SIMPLE PARSLEY TONER FOR OILY SKIN

Parsley is naturally antiseptic and helps to improve circulation, plus it is rich in immune-enhancing vitamins C and A, making it the ideal ingredient for oily skin.

You will need:

½ bunch parsley • 100 ml spring water • 1 teaspoon lemon juice

To prepare:

Roughly chop the parsley into a glass bowl and add the lemon juice. Boil the water and pour over the mixture. Allow to infuse until cool. Pour the mixture through a fine sieve over a glass bottle, then store in the fridge.

To use:

After cleansing, use a quality cotton ball and swipe a generous amount of the toner all over skin, avoiding the eye area. Use night and morning – and throughout the day during hot summer months.

CAMOMILE LIGHTENING HAIR TREATMENT

A gentle lightening treatment that intensifies with exposure to the sun to give your hair a hint of summer.

You will need:

500 ml very strong camomile tea • 125 ml very strong calendula tea • glass pump dispenser bottle • 125 ml fresh lemon juice

To prepare:

Brew the camomile and calendula teas for 30 minutes. Strain the liquid into the pump dispenser bottle together with the fresh lemon juice. Shake to mix thoroughly.

To use:

Spritz the solution onto clean, dry hair, applying the liquid only to the areas to be highlighted. Be sure to thoroughly saturate for best results. For a natural, sun-kissed look, coat the hair ends with the lemon mix. Allow it to absorb for 1 to 2 hours before washing hair thoroughly.

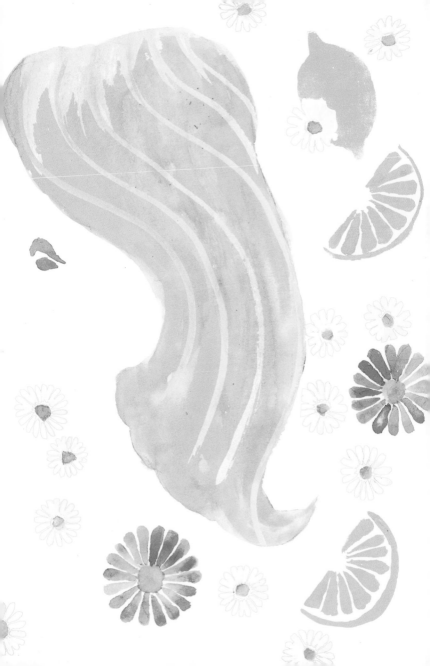

GENTLE ROSE WATER TONER

This beautifully gentle toner is perfect for sensitive skin. Rose water is incredibly cooling and soothing, making it the perfect way to refresh tired skin.

You will need:

3 large handfuls of fresh rose petals, washed • ice cubes

To prepare:

You will need a large pan with a rounded lid, and the pan needs to be large enough for you to place a heatproof bowl inside it, and then put the pan lid on upside down.

Ideally the bowl should not touch the bottom of the pan, so you will need something to act as a pedestal for the bowl to stand on, such as a smaller heatproof pan, dish or ramekin (or something heavy of a similar size).

Place the rose petals into the large pan around the pedestal, place the heatproof bowl on the pedestal and add just enough cold water to cover the petals.

Put the pan lid on upside down (if you only have a flat lid you can use a stainless steel bowl instead – it should be large enough to seal it but shallow enough so that its bottom does not touch the other bowl).

Turn up the heat to bring the water to a boil. Add the ice cubes into the inverted lid. As the rose-infused steam hits the underside of the cold lid, it will condense and drop into the internal bowl.

Turn the heat down and leave simmering gently for 2 to 4 hours. Every now and again, carefully lift the lid and take out a little distilled rose water, stopping when the rose scent of the liquid begins to weaken. Replace the ice and boiling water if needs be as you do this, and do not let the water boil dry.

To use:

Store in a small glass spray bottle. Keep in the fridge and use as need be for extra cooling on the skin.

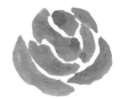

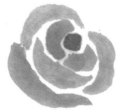

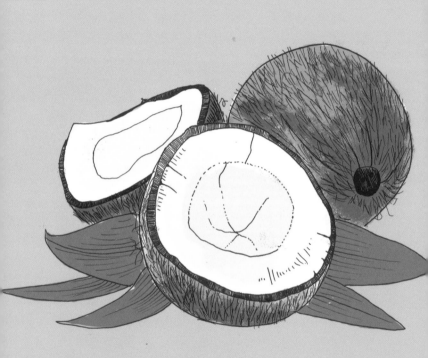

COCONUT

Coconut oil is not only a superfood but also super nourishing on your skin, keeping it hydrated, reducing the appearance of lines and gently exfoliating dead skin cells, making it ideal for keeping even sensitive skin beautifully smooth.

SEA SALT SKIN BUFFER

The combination of sea salt and coconut oil gently polishes your skin to leave it smooth and hydrated.

You will need:

4 tablespoons coconut oil • 2 tablespoons sea salt flakes • 5 drops of essential oil, choose from: peppermint, to invigorate and refresh; citrus, to brighten; lavender, to soothe and calm; • glass jar with lid

To prepare:

Combine the coconut oil and sea salt, mixing thoroughly. Add your essential oil to scent, then use straightaway.

To use:

Massage the skin buffer all over the body. Take care to massage more gently across the delicate décolleté and neck areas. Rinse in a warm shower and gently pat dry. Store in a glass jar in the fridge.

INTENSIVE DRY SKIN BALM

This intensive skin treatment is rich and nourishing for the driest skin. Use on the face and the body.

You will need:

15 ml beeswax pellets • 30 ml sweet almond oil • 30 ml coconut oil • 1 teaspoon rosehip oil • 1 vitamin E capsule • 8 drops of lavender oil • glass jar with lid

To prepare:

Place the pellets, almond, coconut and rosehip oil into a heatproof bowl. Break open and add the vitamin E capsule. Melt over a pan of hot water, then add the lavender oil. Remove from heat and use a hand blender to mix thoroughly. Keep blending the mixture as it cools until it thickens to a light and creamy texture.

To use:

When completely cool, spoon into the jar. Use as an emergency treatment or as a regular face or body moisturizer. Store in a glass jar in the fridge.

LOVELY LEGS SHAVING BALM

These nutrient-rich ingredients will moisturize skin, while the Castile soap results in silky-smooth skin.

You will need:

3 tablespoons coconut oil • 3 tablespoons shea butter
• 2 tablespoons jojoba oil • 2 tablespoons liquid Castile soap
• glass jar with lid

To prepare:

Melt the coconut oil and shea butter in a glass bowl over a pan of hot water. Add the jojoba oil and mix before removing from the heat. Leave to cool and place in the fridge to set. Once solid, leave to soften slightly and break up with a spoon, then blend with a hand blender until the mixture becomes light and fluffy. Add the liquid Castile soap and combine. Spoon the mixture into the glass jar and store in the fridge.

To use:

Massage the balm into the skin to help the shaving blade glide easily over legs, underarms, face and even the bikini line.

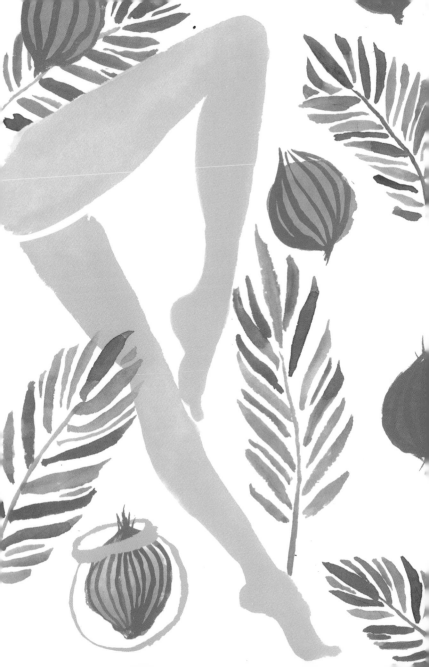

Hydrating Aloe Hair Mist

Coconut water is a delicious tropical hydrator packed with cell-regenerating and anti-ageing cytokinins for plump, soft skin and healthy hair.

You will need:

25 ml coconut water • 25 ml aloe vera juice • 1 vitamin E capsule • 1 teaspoon sweet almond oil • 1 teaspoon macadamia oil

To prepare:

Mix the coconut water and aloe vera juice in a small (100 ml) glass spritz bottle. Break open and add the contents of the vitamin E capsule, the almond oil and macadamia oil. Shake gently to mix.

To use:

After shampooing, spritz all over hair paying particular attention to split ends. Also great to refresh dry hair on long summer days or to rehydrate hair in air-conditioned or heated rooms.

MOISTURIZING COCONUT OIL TREATMENT

This treatment is great for the colder months when skin appears dry and dull.

You will need:

3 tablespoons coconut oil • 1 tablespoon cocoa or shea butter • 10–12 drops of lavender oil • glass jar with lid

To prepare:

Scoop the coconut oil into a glass bowl and add the cocoa or shea butter. Place the glass bowl into a pan of boiling water to melt the mixture. Combine the ingredients well, then remove the bowl from the heat. Add the lavender oil and stir thoroughly as the mixture starts to cool. Pour into the glass jar and leave to cool before fitting the lid. This will keep for up to a week in the fridge.

To use:

Use three times a week for dry to sensitive skin or once a week for oily or acne-prone skin.

HAND AND FOOT SPA TREATMENT

Nourishing, naturally anti-bacterial and anti-fungal coconut oil, mineral-rich sea salt and astringent, whitening lemon makes this the perfect polishing treatment to keep your feet and nails looking great all year long.

You will need:

2 tablespoons coconut oil • 1 tablespoon sea salt • 1 teaspoon lemon juice

To prepare:

Spoon the coconut oil into a glass bowl, add the sea salt and the freshly squeezed lemon juice and combine with a spatula until evenly mixed. Make fresh each time.

To use:

Soak hands and feet in warm water before gently massaging with the spa treatment to remove dry skin, freshen and moisturize. Add a little more pressure when massaging around the nail areas to neaten and moisturize cuticles and whiten and hydrate nails.

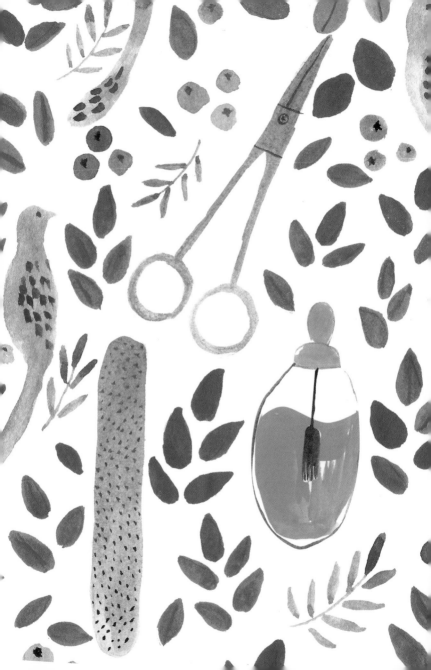

BEETROOT LIP TINT

A natural colour for lips and cheeks, this lip tint will add a hint of pretty pink and keep lips hydrated throughout the day.

You will need:
½ fresh raw beetroot • 1 tablespoon coconut oil • 1 vitamin E capsule • small pots with lids

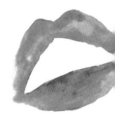

To prepare:
Peel the beetroot and cut it into quarters. Add the coconut oil to a glass bowl, break open and add the vitamin E capsule, then add one piece of beetroot. Place the glass bowl over a pan of simmering water to heat the ingredients and encourage the beetroot juice to flow. Remove the beetroot piece when you are happy with the colour – or add more pieces to create a darker shade. Allow the mixture to cool, then pour into small pots.

To use:
Refrigerate in between uses: the tint will solidify in the fridge but will melt on the lips to leave a pretty, natural hint of colour.

SHEA BUTTER FOOT BALM

A good foot massage is an essential part of a home pedicure regime – but is great at any time to reinvigorate mind, body and soul! This treatment will make feet feel fresh and restored.

You will need:

4 tablespoons coconut oil • 3 tablespoons shea butter • 8 drops of essential oil, choose from: rosemary; spearmint; camomile; lavender • glass jar with lid

To prepare:

Melt the coconut oil with the shea butter in a glass bowl over a pan of simmering water. Remove from the heat and add your chosen essential oil. Pour into a glass jar and store out of direct sunlight.

To use:

Scoop up a generous amount and smother each foot for a nourishing treatment. For very cracked heels, apply the balm and then wear thin, white cotton socks overnight.

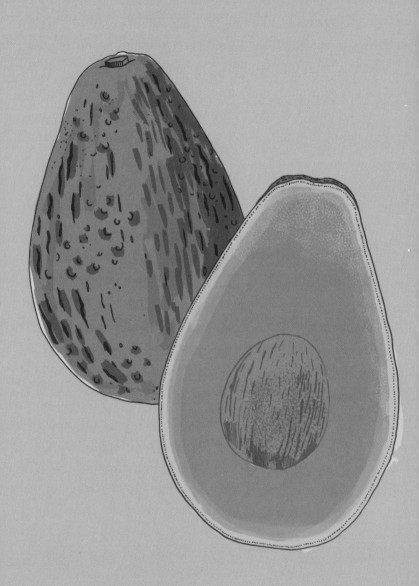

GREENS

Take inspiration from your summer salads, avocado smoothies and detox juices and discover that the power of greens can be just as beneficial to your complexion when enjoyed in these beauty recipes as they are when consumed.

CUCUMBER EYE MASK

The skin around the eye area is fine and delicate, and can be easily irritated by the environment. When your eyes are feeling sore an eye mask offers instant relief. This treatment is hydrating and soothing to help reduce puffiness and restore your natural sparkle.

You will need:

1 teaspoon almond oil • 2 tablespoons grated cucumber

To prepare:

Mix the almond oil with the grated cucumber in a small bowl.

To use:

Apply one tablespoon of the mixture to each closed eye, lie back and relax. Leave for at least 5 minutes before washing off with cool water and gently patting dry. Make fresh each time.

AVOCADO AND OLIVE OIL SERUM

Rich in vitamins and fatty acids, avocado oil melts into the skin to nourish and hydrate. Olive oil contains squalene which locks in moisture. Both oils are high in antioxidants to give a youthful boost to skin.

You will need:

2 tablespoons avocado oil • 2 tablespoons extra virgin olive oil

To prepare:

Pour both oils into a small glass dropper bottle – amber or blue glass will protect the oils from oxidizing in sunlight.

To use:

After cleansing, stir the serum using the dropper then place four drops into the palm of the hand. Lightly massage all over the face until the serum is absorbed. Use morning and night. Apply a little more in colder weather for an extra boost.

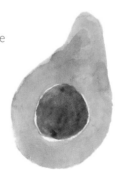

COOLING CUCUMBER TONER FOR SENSITIVE SKIN

Cucumber reduces puffiness and redness. Camomile is also an excellent soothing ingredient – it is an ideal ingredient to use if your skin is super sensitive.

You will need:

1 cucumber • ½ carrot • ¼ cup camomile tea • ½ cup lemon juice

To prepare:

Juice the cucumber and carrot, then add camomile tea and lemon juice . Combine all the ingredients in a glass jar and shake to blend.

To use:

Use a cotton wool ball to apply to your face. Keep refrigerated and store for no longer than three days.

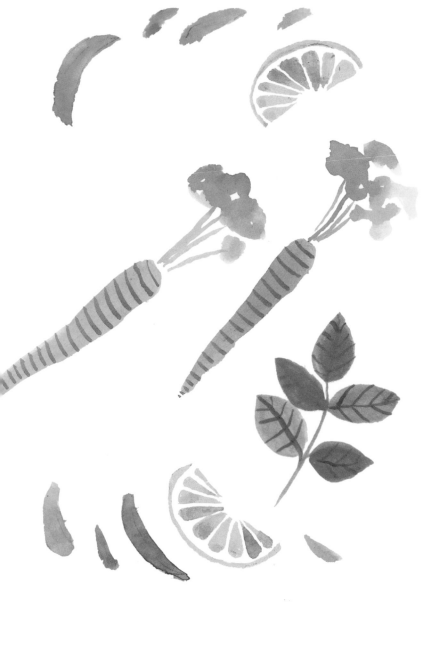

ALOE VERA MOISTURIZER

This moisturizer is for normal to dry skin. For more oily skin, use a ratio of two-thirds aloe vera gel with one-third coconut oil, plus three drops of your essential oil to form a more lotion-type consistency.

You will need:
100 ml aloe vera gel • 200 ml coconut oil • 10 drops of rose or lavender essential oil • glass jar with lid

To prepare:
Blend the aloe vera gel with the coconut oil in a blender. Add your chosen essential oil and then blend again. Pour into an airtight glass jar and store in the fridge.

To use:
The moisturizer will solidify when chilled, so warm a small scoop of it in your palm before smoothing all over the body to moisturize and hydrate skin.

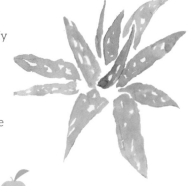

AVOCADO, HONEY AND BANANA FACE MASK

Good enough to eat, the deep moisturising and smoothing properties of banana along with vitamin- and mineral-rich avocado and nourishing honey create a magical mask to soothe and condition skin, leaving it plumped and glowing.

You will need:

½ ripe avocado • ½ ripe banana • 1 teaspoon honey • 1 teaspoon rose water

To prepare:

In a glass bowl, mash the avocado and banana together to form a paste. Add the honey and rose water and combine well.

To use:

Use immediately, smoothing the paste over clean skin with fingertips, avoiding the eye area, then leave for 10 minutes to achieve the very best results. Tissue away residue then rinse with warm water and pat dry.

AVOCADO HAIR THICKENING TREATMENT

This protein-rich treatment mix promotes lustrous hair growth and volume. Avocado is a superfruit, packed with vitamins A, B6, D and E plus magnesium, folic acid, amino acids, copper and iron, which promote thick hair growth.

You will need:
½ avocado • 1 egg white• 2 teaspoons of honey •½ teaspoon wheatgerm oil • 6 drops of rosemary essential oil

To prepare:
Mash the avocado (use whole fruit for long hair) and all the other ingredients to a smooth pulp.

To use:
Apply to your scalp and damp hair, and wrap with either plastic wrap or a shower cap and a warm towel. Leave to absorb for 30 minutes. Shampoo the treatment out, then condition and style as normal. Repeat weekly for visible results.

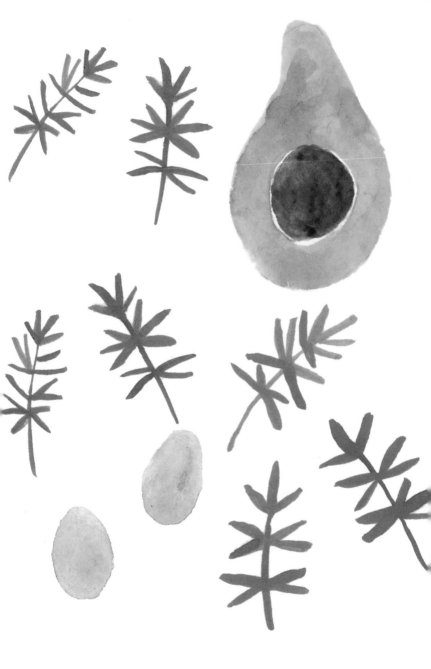

CUCUMBER EYE BAG BLITZ

Bags under the eyes can be a result of too much time in front of a screen, too much or too little sleep or environmental stresses. No matter the cause, this recipe will help to blitz the puffy appearance of eye bags while hydrating the skin.

You will need:

2 cucumber slices • ½ teaspoon coconut oil

To use:

Massage the coconut oil around each eye in a gentle, circular motion, starting at the top inner corner of the eye and sweeping around the eye socket to finish at the bottom corner.

Repeat the massage strokes several times, then place a cucumber slice over each eye and relax for 10 minutes. Repeat every evening, if you can, to keep eye bags at bay.

COLLAGEN-BOOSTING MOISTURIZER

A small amount of this luxury moisturizer goes a long way! This rich moisturizer can be used both morning and night.

You will need:
2 teaspoons shea butter • 1 teaspoon almond oil • 1 teaspoon avocado oil • 4 tablespoons spring water • 1 tablespoons emulsifying wax • 1 teaspoon glycerine • 1 teaspoon honey

To prepare:
Combine the shea butter, almond and avocado oils in a glass bowl over hot water and stir until the butter has melted. Remove from the heat but keep warm with a cloth cover. Heat the spring water to 80 degrees Celsius (175 degrees Fahrenheit) then add the emulsifying wax, glycerin and honey, stirring until dissolved. Remove from the heat then combine all ingredients into the pan and whisk until smooth. Allow to cool before placing in a storage jar. Keep in the fridge.

To use:
Warm a pea-sized amount between the fingertips then massage into skin, taking care to avoid the eye area.

REJUVENATING CUCUMBER FACE AND BODY MIST

Soothe and enliven both face and body with this refreshing, mineral-rich mist. Cucumber cleanses and hydrates, improving the complexion of your skin and restoring your natural glow.

You will need:

2 cucumbers • cotton muslin cloth • 80 ml rose water • 100 ml capacity spray bottle

To prepare:

Wash the cucumbers and finely grate them into a glass bowl. Strain the mixture through the muslin cloth into a second glass bowl to extract the cucumber water. Combine with the rose water, then pour into the spray bottle.

To use:

Spray over the face and body to condition and cool skin throughout the hot summer months.

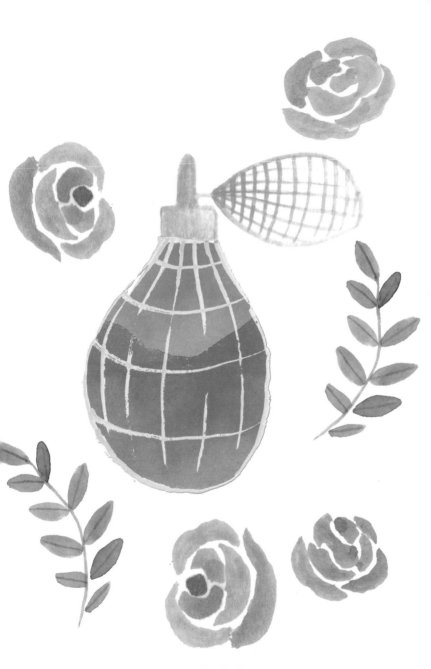

CASTER SUGAR FACE POLISH FOR SENSITIVE SKIN

Avocados are great for sensitive and dry skin, containing monosaturated fats, potassium, phosphorus, calcium and A, B, C and E vitamins.

You will need:

½ avocado • 2 tablespoons caster sugar

To prepare:

Mash the avocado in a glass bowl and add the caster sugar, mixing thoroughly. Add a little more caster sugar to make a thicker paste if required.

To use:

Gently massage the paste over the face for a few minutes, avoiding the eye area, and then leave on for a further 5 minutes to maximize the benefits of the avocado oils. Tissue off then rinse in cool water.

LETTUCE, CUCUMBER AND GREEN TEA TONER

The vitamins, phosphorus and silicon found in lettuce combine perfectly with the vitamin C and high water content of cucumber to make this antioxidant-rich toner.

You will need:

1 green tea teabag • ½ lettuce • ½ cucumber (peeled)

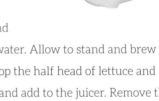

To prepare:

Place the green tea teabag into a glass bowl and pour over 100 ml boiling water. Allow to stand and brew for 5 minutes. Roughly chop the half head of lettuce and the peeled half cucumber and add to the juicer. Remove the green tea teabag from the brewed, cooled tea and add the lettuce and cucumber juice.

To use:

Use straightaway or pour into a glass bottle with a tight-fitting cap and then store in the fridge.

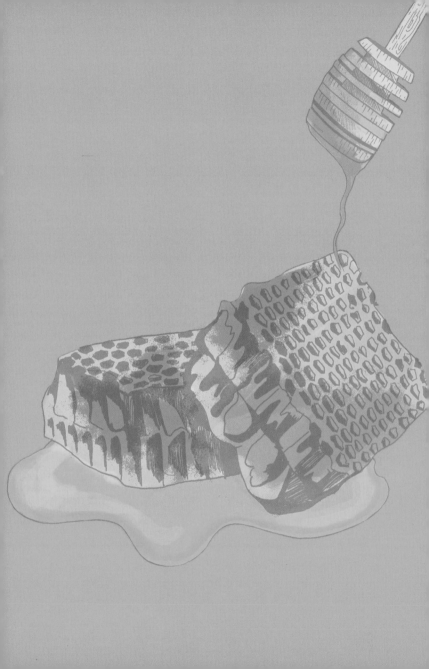

HONEY

Honey is a wonderful ingredient that can give your complexion the boost it needs to regain its natural glow. Full of antioxidants, naturally antibacterial and clarifying, it will give you beautifully soft and younger looking hair and nails.

BEESWAX MOISTURIZER

Choose whether to add essential oils, such as ylang ylang (for smooth skin), geranium (to revitalize) or camomile (to calm and soothe).

You will need:
glass jar with lid • beeswax beads or pellets • olive oil • almond oil • 4 vitamin E capsules • 10 drops of essential oil (optional)

To prepare:
Fill the glass jar one-quarter full with the beeswax and fill the remaining three-quarters with equal quantities of olive oil and almond oil. Stand the glass jar in a pan of hot water and stir until the mixture melts. Remove and allow to cool to room temperature, stirring occasionally. Break open the vitamin E capsules and add to the mixture together with your chosen essential oil, stirring until combined.

To use:
The moisturizer is ready to use when cool. It is ideal for when your skin is feeling dry. Store in a cool, dark place.

HONEY AND LEMON FACIAL CLEANSER

The healing power of honey is perfect for all skin types including oily, acne-prone, dry and ageing skin. Honey's natural antiseptic qualities make this an ideal cleanser for rosacea and dark spots.

You will need:

2 tablespoons honey • 1 tablespoon lemon juice

To prepare:

Simply combine in a glass bowl.

To use:

After cleansing, massage the mixture into the skin, taking care to avoid the eye area. It may feel tingly as the lemon juice starts to take effect. Tissue away any residue then rinse face in warm water. Skin will feel clean and refreshed. This recipe can also be applied as a mask 2 to 3 times a week for best results.

ARGAN FACIAL MOISTURIZER

This moisturizer is ideal for dry or mature skin or for those colder months when your skin needs an extra moisture boost.

You will need:

1 teaspoon shea butter • 2 teaspoon argan oil • 1 teaspoon avocado oil • 1 teaspoon beeswax • 4 tablespoons spring water • 1 teaspoon honey • 1 tablespoon emulsifying wax • 1 teaspoon glycerin

To prepare:

Place the shea butter, argan and avocado oils together with the beeswax into a glass bowl over hot water. Stir gently until the butter and wax are melted, remove from the heat but keep warm with a cloth cover. Heat the spring water to 80 degrees Celsius (175 degrees Fahrenheit) then add the emulsifying wax, glycerin and honey. Stir until completely dissolved. Remove from the heat then add the hot oil mixture to the pan. Whisk the mixture with a hand-held whisk or stick blender to create a smooth cream. Allow to cool, taking care to stir occasionally, then pour into a glass jar and store in the fridge.

BROWN SUGAR LIP SCRUB

As brown sugar has smaller particles than sea salt, it is a more gentle option to keep sensitive areas such as the lips soft, flake-free and smooth and always ready for a pop of colour.

You will need:

1 teaspoon brown sugar • 1 tablespoon organic coconut oil • 1 teaspoon honey

To prepare:

Spoon all ingredients into a glass bowl and mix until thoroughly combined. Add a little more brown sugar if you prefer a thicker lip scrub.

To use:

Gently massage a pea-sized amount of the scrub into your lips to loosen rough, flaky skin and to nourish and condition. Rinse away any residue to leave plump and soft lips. Best used at night. To store, spoon the mixture into a small glass pot with a lid and store in the fridge.

HONEY HAIR CONDITIONER

Honey is the perfect conditioning agent for hair – its natural humectant properties mean moisture is locked into the hair shaft, so hair feels soft and looks smooth and glossy.

You will need:

1 tablespoon shea butter • 1 tablespoon coconut oil • 1 tablespoon argan oil • 1 teaspoon honey

To prepare:

Spoon all ingredients into a glass bowl over hot water and mix continuously until the butter melts. Remove from the heat and allow to cool for 30 minutes. Using a hand-held whisk or stick blender whisk the mixture continuously to form a thick yoghurt consistency. Allow to cool thoroughly and spoon into a glass jar with a lid. Store in the fridge.

To use:

Before shampooing, scoop a coin-sized amount and massage through damp hair, concentrating on the ends and scalp. Wrap hair in a warm towel and leave for 30 to 40 minutes. Rinse and then gently shampoo hair to remove residue.

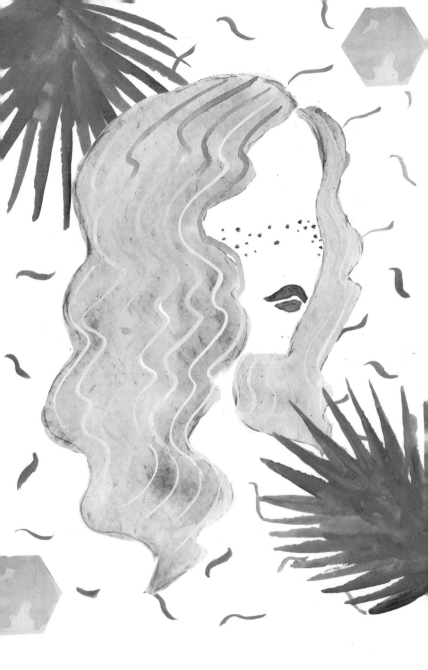

HONEY AND SHEA BUTTER LIP BALM

The super-moisturising, vitamin-packed, skin-protecting properties of shea butter and beeswax make this the ideal lip balm for windy or wintry days. The added castor oil helps to heal while the honey soothes dry, flaky lips.

You will need:

1 tablespoon shea butter • 1 teaspoon castor oil • 1 teaspoon sunflower oil • 1 teaspoon beeswax • ¼ teaspoon honey • glass jar with lid

To prepare:

Place all ingredients into a glass bowl and stand over hot water until the beeswax is melted. Stir well to combine all the ingredients then remove from the heat. Allow to cool then pour into a glass jar with a lid.

To use:

Apply as required to dry lips or at bedtime as a nightly treat to condition and nourish.

AVOCADO AND HONEY COMPLEXION POLISH

The perfect recipe to revitalize dull, tired complexions, this gentle skin polish harnesses the natural exfoliating and soothing powers of honey to leave skin soft and moisturized.

You will need:

½ ripe avocado • 1 teaspoon honey • 1 tablespoon olive oil • 1 tablespoon ground rice

To prepare:

Spoon the honey and olive oil into a glass bowl and warm over hot water. Remove from the heat then mash the avocado and add to the bowl. Mix well before stirring in the ground rice to form a smooth paste.

To use:

Apply immediately to clean skin, massaging gently over the face, especially around areas of congestion. Leave for 2 minutes, then rinse with warm water and pat dry.

RICE WATER, HONEY AND ROSE WATER CLEANSING LOTION

This hydrating lotion is great for cleansing, soothing and moisturising both mature skins and acne-prone skin.

You will need:
5 tablespoons rice (any type) • spring water • 2 teaspoons honey • 1 tablespoon rose water

To prepare:
Rinse the rice in cold water then place into a bowl and pour over 1 cup of spring water and leave standing for 45 minutes to release the vitamins and minerals. Stir thoroughly and then strain the water with a sieve over a glass storage jar. Add the honey and stir thoroughly, then add the rose water.

To use:
Pour a little of the lotion onto a soft cotton ball and swipe all over the face to remove dirt and impurities. Apply a second time until the cotton ball is clean. Skin will feel refreshed with a radiant glow. Use morning and night.

HONEY, NUTMEG AND CINNAMON BLEMISH CONTROL

The power-blend of detoxifying and antimicrobial nutmeg and cinnamon help unclog pores while the anti-inflammatory, healing properties of honey help keep blemishes at bay.

You will need:

1 teaspoon honey • ½ teaspoon nutmeg

• ½ teaspoon cinnamon

To prepare:

Place all ingredients into a small glass and mix thoroughly.

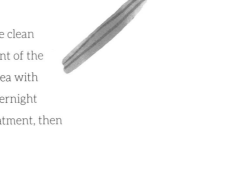

To use:

Ensure face and hands are clean and smooth a small amount of the mixture to the affected area with the fingertip. Leave on overnight for the most effective treatment, then rinse and cleanse.

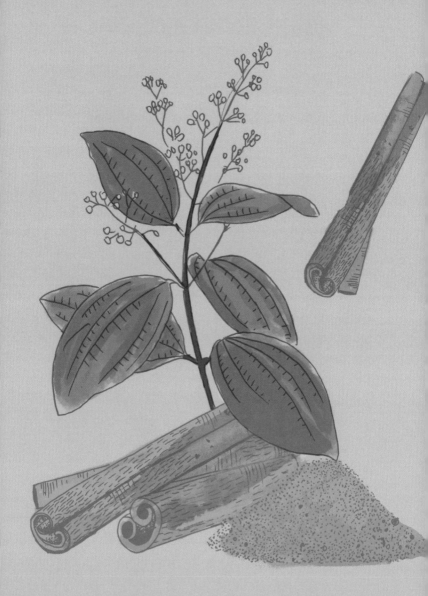

SUGAR, SODA & SPICE

From creating your own dry shampoo with bicarbonate of soda to mixing your own make-up with cornflour, these dry cupboard staples go way beyond the kitchen. These ingredients protect and nourish, invigorate and soothe, allowing you to benefit from them whatever your mood.

CINNAMON LIP BALM

Lips have no oil glands and have very thin skin, so they need extra care to keep them soft, supple and kissable! This plumping balm will keep your lips smooth and hydrated.

You will need:

3 tablespoons coconut oil • 2 tablespoons beeswax pellets • 2 vitamin E capsules • ½ teaspoon honey • 12 drops of cinnamon essential oil

To prepare:

Mix the coconut oil and beeswax pellets in a glass bowl over a pan of simmering water until melted. Remove from heat, break open and add the vitamin E capsules to the bowl together with the honey and cinnamon oil. Mix thoroughly and pour into a small pot to harden.

TURMERIC TEETH WHITENER

The bicarbonate of soda acts as a mild abrasive to rid teeth of stains, while its alkaline properties help to neutralize acids and bacteria. Coconut oil works to reduce bacteria and promotes healthy gums, while the turmeric has important anti-inflammatory properties.

You will need:

3 tablespoons ground turmeric • 2 teaspoons bicarbonate of soda • 2 tablespoons coconut oil • glass jar with lid

To prepare:

Combine the turmeric with the bicarbonate of soda. Add the coconut oil, then mix thoroughly and spoon into a glass jar.

To use:

Use a pea-sized amount on a clean toothbrush and brush your teeth in a soft, circular motion for 3 minutes, then rinse and spit several times. Although the turmeric is yellow your teeth will be shining white! Store in a glass jar in the fridge.

SUGAR BODY SCRUB

Bring the luxury of a spa treatment into your everyday life with this deliciously indulgent body scrub.

You will need:

250 g brown sugar • 250 ml avocado oil • 2 teaspoons aloe vera gel • 2 drops of lavender essential oil

To prepare:

Combine all the ingredients in a bowl.

To use:

Scoop some of the scrub out using your hand and massage gently onto your skin for a minute (the scrub will tighten onto your skin like a mask). Leave on for 3 to 4 minutes before rinsing. The scrub can be used all over your body and is suitable for most skin types. If you don't have the above ingredients, you can just add sugar to any cleanser for a moisturising, exfoliating scrub for smooth

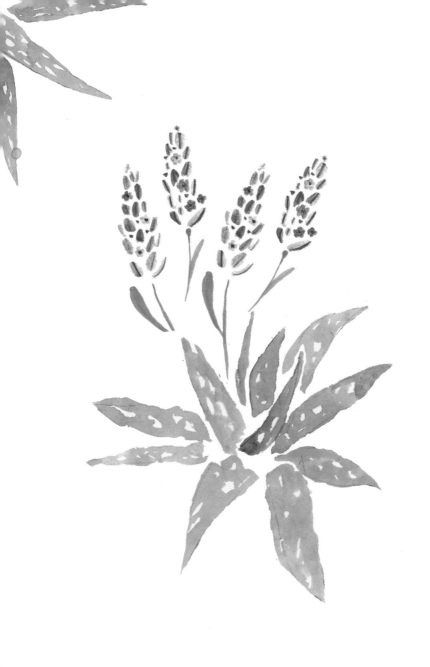

BICARBONATE OF SODA DRY SHAMPOO

This dry shampoo will leave hair looking and smelling fresh with the added benefit of adding volume and lift to fine hair.

You will need:

4 tablespoons cornflour • 1 tablespoon bicarbonate of soda • glass jar with lid

To prepare:

Combine the cornflour and bicarbonate of soda in the glass jar and shake vigorously to combine the ingredients.

To use:

To apply, pinch a small amount between fingers and sprinkle along the hairline. Massage through hair to allow the mixture to grab any excess oil, then brush through to remove the residue.

For easy application, spoon the dry shampoo into a clean spice jar with a perforated top.

CINNAMON BATH SALTS

With natural anti-microbials, anti-fungal and purifying properties, stimulating cinnamon help improve circulation and the health of skin and when added to magnesium-rich Epsom salts or mineral-laden sea salt, creates a warming bath that leaves you feeling calm and comfortable. Perfect to encourage restful sleep at bed time.

You will need:

100 g Epsom salts or sea salt • 2 tablespoons fine cinnamon powder • 1 teaspoon vanilla essence (alcohol-free)

To prepare:

Pour the Epsom salts or sea salt into a glass bowl then add the fine cinnamon powder and mix thoroughly. Sprinkle the vanilla essence over the mixture then combine quickly to ensure even distribution throughout the bath salts.

To use:

Just a handful of these bath salts poured into a running bath will create a wonderful uplifting fragrance and a lovely, warming and relaxing bath.

CACAO EYEBROW THICKENER

The eyebrows create a perfect frame for the face and the following recipe will help keep them full and healthy.

You will need:

1 teaspoon cornflour • ½ teaspoon cacao powder (unsweetened) • small pot with lid • cotton buds

To prepare:

Combine the cornflour and cacao powder and use a cotton bud to gently brush over the brows and blend. If eyebrows are dark, add more cacao powder to intensify the colour. Store in a small pot.

To use:

For an extra treatment at night time, swipe a little almond oil over brows to encourage healthy growth.

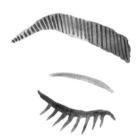

BAKING SODA DEODORANT

Keep odour and moisture free with this easy deodorant. The coconut oil base will help keep odour-causing bacteria at bay while nourishing and protecting the delicate underarm area.

You will need:

1-2 tablespoons coconut oil • 3 tablespoons arrowroot • 1 tablespoon baking soda

To prepare:

Spoon the coconut oil into a glass bowl and add the arrowroot and baking soda. Mix to form a stiff paste, adding equal amounts of arrowroot and baking soda as required. Store in a glass jar with a lid.

To use:

Scoop a pea-sized amount with the fingertips to warm the paste and then smooth gently under each arm. Remove any residue with a tissue before dressing.

PEACH, COCONUT OIL AND BROWN SUGAR BODY SCRUB

Peaches are rich in alpha hydroxy acid AHA, a natural and gentle skin exfoliant, which breaks down dead skin cells and encourages fresh cell turnover.

You will need:

2 ripe peaches • 1 tablespoon coconut or almond oil • 1 tablespoon honey • 2 tablespoons brown sugar

To prepare:

Peel the peaches then place in a glass bowl and puree with a stick blender until smooth. Stir in the oil, honey and brown sugar until combined.

To use:

Massage all over the body with fingertips in a circular motion in upward and downward strokes – always towards the heart. Allow the scrub to sit on the skin for 5 minutes before rinsing gently with a warm washcloth. Skin will look polished and feel silky smooth.

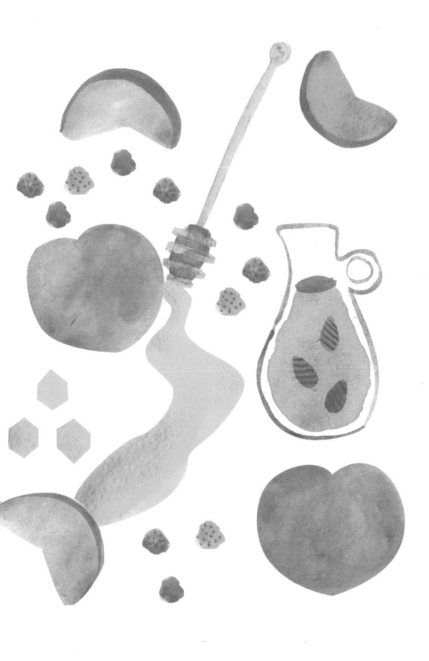

BLACK PEPPER, CAMOMILE AND COCONUT SCALP BALM

Black pepper, a surprising source of vitamins A and C, will help to increase blood flow to the hair follicles while the nourishing coconut oil moisturizes the scalp to produce a wonderfully warming balm to stimulate hair growth.

You will need:

1 tablespoon coconut oil • 1 teaspoon finely ground black pepper • 4 drops camomile oil

To prepare:

Spoon coconut oil into a glass bowl then finely grind the black pepper using a mortar and pestle. Add the ground black pepper and four drops of camomile oil and blend thoroughly.

To use:

Before shampooing hair, gently massage the balm into the scalp then wrap hair in a warm towel for 30 minutes. Rinse with clear water then shampoo to remove any residue.

GINGER AND MINT HAIR RINSE

The combination of invigorating ginger and refreshing mint helps stimulate blood circulation and balance the pH of the scalp, which in turn encourages hair growth and condition. Hair is healthier and shiny with a lovely, fresh scent.

You will need:

4 cm root ginger • small bunch fresh mint • 100 ml spring water

To prepare:

Grate the root ginger into a glass bowl then add the finely chopped mint. Boil the spring water then pour over the ingredients and allow to infuse until cool. Strain the liquid through a fine sieve into a glass jar with a lid.

To use:

After every hair wash, pour a little of the hair rinse through the hair and massage into the scalp. Store in the fridge.

CLOVE AND BICARBONATE OF SODA TOOTHPASTE

Baking soda is a great odour absorber, leaving teeth and mouth feeling super fresh and clean. The toothpaste can be used either in solid or liquid form.

You will need:

2 tablespoons of coconut oil • 1 tablespoon of bicarbonate of soda • 5 whole cloves • small glass jar with lid

To prepare:

Grind the whole cloves into a fine powder using a pestle and mortar. Spoon the coconut oil into a glass bowl, then add the baking soda and ground cloves. Mix thoroughly and spoon into a small glass jar with a lid.

To use:

Add a little of the mixture to the soft toothbrush and gently work around your teeth and gums in a circular motion. Swish the mixture around your mouth to allow bacteria and debris to be absorbed by the baking soda. Spit out the mixture and debris – try not to swallow!

TURMERIC, LEMON AND YOGHURT FACE MASK

Rich in antioxidants, and anti-inflammatory benefits, turmeric can help even out pigmentation and calm skin to achieve a more youthful glow.

You will need:

½ teaspoon turmeric • 1 tablespoon natural yoghurt • ½ teaspoon lemon juice

To prepare:

Spoon the natural yogurt into a glass bowl then add the turmeric and lemon juice and mix thoroughly.

To use:

Spread a thin layer all over the face, taking care to avoid the eye area.
Leave for up to 15 minutes then gently tissue off before cleansing thoroughly. Skin will look and feel fresh, ready for moisturising. Try this mask once a month to maintain benefits.

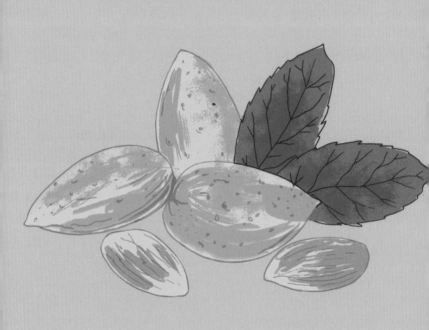

NUTS, GRAINS & SEEDS

From protein-rich flaxseed for nourishing nails, oats for calming irritated skin, and walnuts for a natural hair colourant, these nuts, grain and seed recipes will have you glowing from head to toe!

SOOTHING OATMEAL SOAK

The base of oats is soothing and moisturising, and will help to reduce itching and soreness, while the essential oils are calming for your nerves, helping to promote relaxation.

You will need:

2 tablespoons rolled oats • 2 x 15 cm squares of natural muslin (or a ready-made spice bag) • cotton thread • needle • 1 tablespoon milk powder • 3 vitamin E capsules

To prepare:

If making your own bag, sew together the two squares of muslin, leaving one side open. In a glass bowl, mix the milk powder and the rolled oats. Break open and add the vitamin E capsules. Combine thoroughly, then spoon into the muslin bag and sew along the top edge (or close by tying drawstrings on the ready-made bag).

To use:

Drop the bag into the running bath water, leave to infuse in the bath and relax.

ALMOND BUTTER CREAM

Ideal for pregnant women, but also anyone who suffers from stretch marks.

You will need:

125 g cocoa butter • 1 teaspoon almond oil • 1 teaspoon vitamin E oil

To prepare:

Place all the ingredients in an ovenproof glass container and gently heat in the microwave, or over a pan of boiling water, until the cocoa butter is melted and the oils are well mixed. Pour into a clean container and allow the cream to cool completely. You may need to stir the cream one more time after it has cooled. Store in a container in a cool, dry place.

To use:

Use after showering to maintain moisture.

MID-WEEK GRAINS SCRUB

Using grains ensures that you won't experience a sensitive reaction, as they are quite soft on your skin.

You will need:

2 tablespoons oatmeal • 2 tablespoons cornmeal • 2 tablespoons wheat germ

To prepare:

Perfect for exfoliating normal to sensitive skin. Mix ingredients together and store in an airtight container. Make a paste by adding warm water to 1 tablespoon of the mixture.

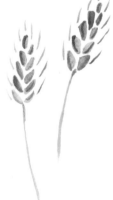

To use:

This recipe is great if you like to exfoliate more than once a week.

CHIA SEED, HONEY AND ROSEMARY ENHANCING FACIAL

Chia seeds are a rich source of skin-loving omega 3 fatty acids, B vitamins, vitamin E plus magnesium and zinc that will help give your complexion a youthful glow.

You will need:

2 tablespoons chia seeds • small sprig rosemary • 1 teaspoon lemon juice • 1 tablespoon honey

To prepare:

Using a pestle and mortar, gently grind the chia seeds to break the outer husk then tip into a small glass bowl. Add the leaves from the rosemary sprig, the lemon juice and the honey and mix thoroughly.

To use:

With clean fingertips, massage all over the face, taking care to avoid the eye area, then leave as a mask for 15 minutes. Gently tissue away residue and rinse skin in cool water. Skin will look and feel noticeably brighter with a fresh radiance.

HAIR GLOSSING TREATMENT

This glossing gel is the perfect de-frizz agent – in one step nourishing and helping to style locks to a sleek, shiny finish. This non-sticky gel is the ultimate natural hair styling product to create a glistening hair texture and frizz-free result.

You will need:

90 ml aloe vera gel • 30 ml jojoba oil • 12 drops of lavender essential oil • 8 drops of sandalwood essential oil • medium dark-glass jar with lid

To prepare:

Mix all the ingredients thoroughly in the dark-glass jar to a smooth gel-like paste.

To use:

Apply the gel sparingly to your hair ends after washing and before blow-drying, and use a small quantity on the fingertips to pull through hair ends.

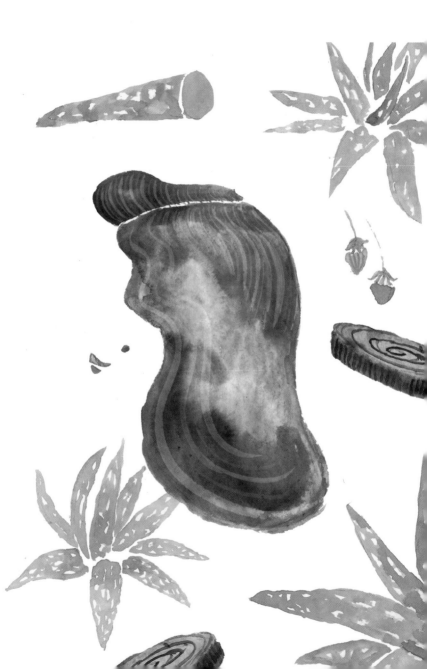

DARKENING HAIR TREATMENT

Walnut powder is a natural colourant that gives wonderful glossy results. It can be bought online or in health-food stores.

You will need:
60 g black walnut powder • small muslin bag • freshly boiled water

To prepare:
Pour the walnut powder into the muslin bag and steep in a bowl containing 1.5 litres of freshly boiled water. Leave for 6 hours or overnight.

To use:
Remove the muslin bag and discard.
Pour the walnut rinse through the hair while showering and comb through. Allow your hair to dry naturally in sunlight, if possible, to create super dark coverage over colour-treated or grey hair. Repeat daily until the desired colour is reached, and fortnightly to retain coverage.

REJUVENATING PEACH, BANANA AND OATMEAL FACE MASK

Banana and peach help to hydrate and rejuvenate dull skin as they are natural sources of folates and lutein, which boost cellular renewal and skin elasticity. Nurturing oatmeal is also great for damaged skin and blemishes.

You will need:
½ peach • 1 banana • 1 tablespoon ground oatmeal

To prepare:
Using a food processor or stick blender, place the peach and banana into a glass bowl and blend to form a fine paste. Add the ground oatmeal and mix well.

To use:
Apply with fingertips over the face and neck, avoiding the eye area. Leave for 20 minutes then rinse off gently with warm water and pat dry. The skin will feel calm and soothed and will look fresh and rejuvenated.

MACADAMIA NUT HAIR HEAT PROTECTOR

This formulation shields hair from the drying effects of any heated appliance, and treats hair with nourishing oils to restore shine and vitality.

You will need:

4 tablespoons macadamia nut oil • 2 tablespoons grapeseed oil • small glass jar with lid

To prepare:

Pour the macadamia nut oil and grapeseed oil into the glass jar and shake to combine.

To use:

Wash and condition your hair as normal, then towel-dry before applying a little of the heat-protection solution to the ends of the hair. Work through to the ends with your fingers before styling. Store away from direct sunlight.

ALMOND, COFFEE AND COCONUT BODY SCRUB

Caffeine is a great stimulant for the circulation and is thought to help in the metabolism of fat deposits.

You will need:

4 tablespoons coconut oil • 1 tablespoon fresh coffee grounds • 2 tablespoons almond meal

To prepare:

Place all the ingredients into a glass bowl and mix thoroughly. For a more intensive cellulite treatment, add an extra ½ tablespoon coffee grounds. If making a batch, spoon the scrub into a glass jar with a lid and store in the fridge.

To use:

Dampen skin under the shower and massage the scrub all over the body in upward sweeps always towards the heart, concentrating on the legs and thighs to help reduce the appearance of cellulite. Shower away the residue.

JOJOBA LASH CONDITIONER

Wearing mascara every day can leave eyelashes dry, brittle and susceptible to breakage. Try giving your eyelashes a weekend break from mascara and replace it with this treatment to strengthen, restore and encourage healthy growth.

You will need:

2 tablespoons jojoba oil • 2 tablespoons aloe vera gel • small pot or jar with lid • cotton buds

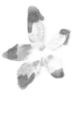

To prepare:

In a small glass bowl mix the jojoba oil and aloe vera gel and pour into the pot.

To use:

Apply with a cotton bud along the base of the lashes, sweeping the length of the lashes, morning and evening, using a fresh cotton bud each time. Store in the fridge.

NATURAL AFTER SUN GEL

Use this soothing anti-inflammatory and super-hydrating treatment to help replenish parched skin.

You will need:

30 ml aloe vera gel • 10 ml jojoba oil • 10 ml sweet almond oil • 10 drops of camomile essential oil • 10 drops of geranium essential oil • 10 drops of lavender essential oil • 2–3 evening primrose oil capsules

To prepare:

In a small glass bowl mix together the aloe vera gel with the jojoba oil, sweet almond oil and the essential oils. Break open the evening primrose oil capsules and add to the bowl. Mix again to combine.

To use:

Gently pat the skin dry and then liberally apply the after-sun mixture all over the body, allowing full absorption. Make fresh each time. Always seek medical help for severe sunburn.

EXFOLIATING VIBRANCY FACIAL SCRUB

Perfect for normal to oily skin, this versatile scrub leaves skin free of dirt and dead cells. The basil helps to lift greying cells and enlivens skin tone for the ultimate spring-clean effect.

You will need:

pinch of salt • ½ teaspoon cider vinegar • 1 drop of basil essential oil • 1 teaspoon ground almonds • 1 teaspoon oat flakes (ground to a rough sand consistency using a pestle and mortar)

To prepare:

Thoroughly mix the salt, vinegar and basil essential oil together in a small bowl, then add the ground almonds and oat flakes.

To use:

Using your fingers, apply the mixture to the face in very gentle circular rolling patterns, focusing on the chin, nose and forehead, and taking care to avoid the eyes.

FLAXSEED NAIL SERUM

Boost cracked cuticles, support weak nails and encourage nail growth with this super nail serum based on flaxseeds, which are rich in protein, fatty acids and calcium.

You will need:

3 tablespoons whole flaxseeds • spring water • 5 drops jojoba oil

To prepare:

Boil the whole flaxseeds in 1 cup of filtered water until it thickens. Strain the mixture through a sieve into a glass bowl and add the jojoba oil, stir and allow to cool. Pour into a small glass jar and store in the fridge.

To use:

Massage the serum into nails and the nail bed and allow to dry. Repeat daily for healthy, strong nails.

NUTTY BODY SCRUB

Using natural ingredients such as nuts and oatmeal will not only exfoliate your body without irritating it, but the oil in the nuts will also provide a moisturising film on your skin, so your skin won't dry out. For all skin types, particularly dry.

You will need:
100 g finely ground nuts (try almonds or flaxseeds)
• 50 g oatmeal • 50 g whole wheat flour

To prepare:
Blend the ingredients until they are reduced to a coarse mixture. Pour into a glass jar with a screw top.

To use:
Scoop out a handful and place into a bowl, adding water to make a paste. Rub over your body to loosen any dry or flaking skin. The mixture can be stored in a freezer.

SHEA NUT BUTTER CUTICLE CREAM

Cuticles should never be cut with scissors. Instead, massage gently with this hydrating cream and push back gently using an orange stick.

You will need:

2 tablespoons shea butter • 1 tablespoon coconut oil • 1 teaspoon beeswax pellets • 7 drops of lavender oil • small glass jar with lid

To prepare:

Melt the shea butter, coconut oil and beeswax pellets in a glass bowl over a pan of simmering water. Store in a small glass jar out of direct sunlight.

To use:

Apply a thin layer of the cream to cuticles and fingertips at night before bed.

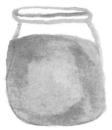

INDEX

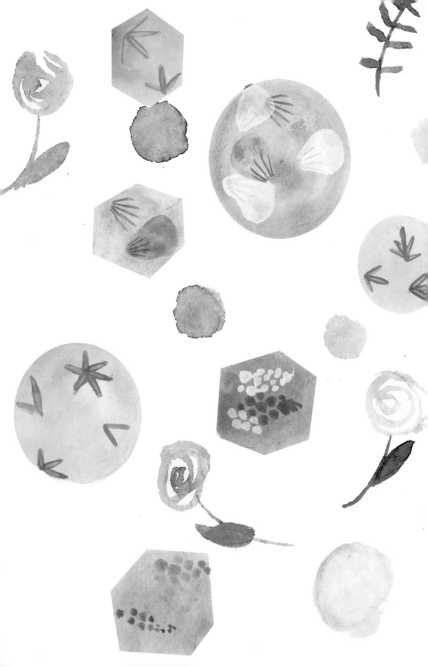